Low-Oxalate Cookbook

Quick and Easy Recipes

Full of Flavour

By

Minna Rose

LionheART Publishing House
Harrogate
UK

www.lionheartgalleries.co.uk
www.facebook.com/lionheartpublishing
publishing@lionheartgalleries.co.uk

First published in Great Britain in 2016 by
LionheART Publishing House

Copyright © Minna Rose 2016
ISBN: 978-1-910115-58-9

Contents

Introduction 1

The Low-Oxalate Kitchen 2

Herbs and Spices 3

1. Salmon with Lime and Honey 4

2. Trout with Apple Stuffing 6

3. Cod in a Garlic, Parsley and White Wine Sauce 8

4. Chicken and Pesto Pasta 10

5. Lemon Chicken 12

6. Mango and Lime Chicken 14

7. Chicken and Ham Pie 16

8. Pork Steaks with a Mustard and Apple Sauce 18

9. Smoked Gammon, Sauerkraut and Bread Dumplings 20

10. Steak with Dijon Mustard Sauce 22

11. Risotto 24

12. Low-Ox Salad 26

13. Pink Salad Dressing 27

14. Vinaigrette 28

15. German Meat Salad 29

16. Vanilla Panna Cotta 30

17. Lemon Pancakes 32

References 34

Food is our body's fuel, and when we are ill, what we eat becomes even more important.

Choosing particular foods and avoiding others can help your body fight your symptoms, and Minna Rose's Cooking for Health series of cookbooks are designed to help you in your quest for better health.

Introduction

Oxalates are organic acids, found in most vegetables and fruits, and which hinder the absorption of calcium. A low-oxalate diet can therefore help people who suffer from osteoporosis and calcium kidney stones to manage their condition. Oxalates may also be a contributing factor in the pain of fibromyalgia, and again a low-oxalate diet may help.

Having suffered from fibromyalgia for many years, Minna Rose has created this 'recipe book for pain', refusing to compromise on flavour and creating delicious meals using only foods low in oxalates.

Fresh and nutritious food is very important for a healthy life, just as tasty food, shared in good company, is essential for a happy and enjoyable life. Minna Rose's cookbooks combine the two in her recipes, all of which are easy to follow and recreate, and accompanied by mouth-watering photography.

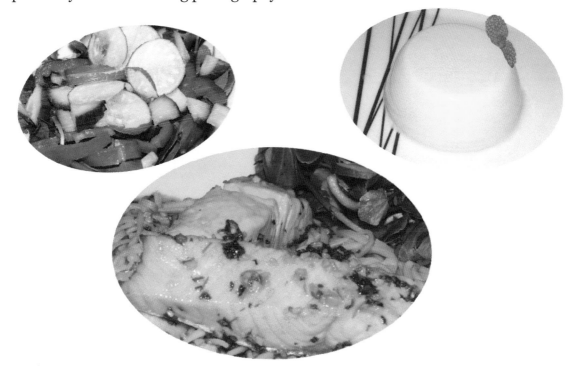

Author's Note:

Because of differences between the imperial measurements used in the UK and US, I have kept all measurements metric to avoid any confusion.

The Low-Oxalate Kitchen

These foods are all low in oxalates:

All meats and fish
Dairy
Eggs
Sugar
White bread
White pasta
White rice

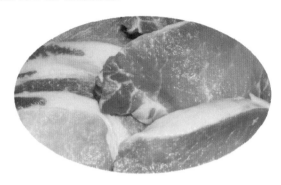

The Low-Oxalate Vegetable Basket

Broccoli (boiled)
Cauliflower
Courgette/Zucchini
Cucumber
Lettuce
Mushroom
Pea
Pumpkin

Radish
Raisin
Red Pepper
Swede
Turnip
Watercress
White Cabbage
White Onion

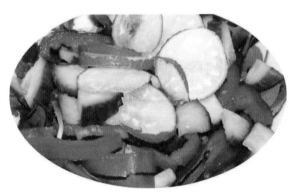 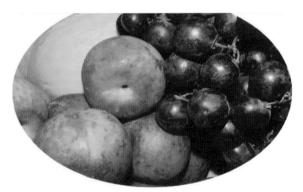

The Low-Oxalate Fruit Bowl

Apple
Apricot
Avocado
Cherry
Coconut
Gherkin
Grape

Lemon
Lime
Melon
Passion fruit
Peach
Pineapple
Plum

Herbs and Spices

One of the hardest things when cooking for a low-oxalate diet is adding flavour. Many spices and other high-flavoured foods are high in oxalates and should be avoided. The following ingredients can add varied and at times intense flavour without adding oxalates, and they are used extensively throughout this cookbook.

Fresh Herbs
To get the most flavour from your herbs, try steeping them in hot water before adding to your dish.

Chives
Coriander leaf (Cilantro)
Dill
Parsley
Rosemary
Tarragon
Thyme

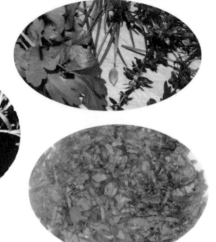

Dried Herbs
Basil

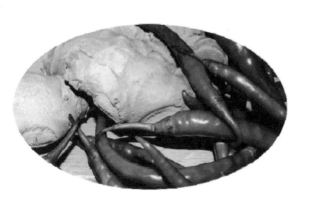

Spices
Fresh ginger
Green Chilli
Cayenne
Nutmeg
Mustard
White pepper

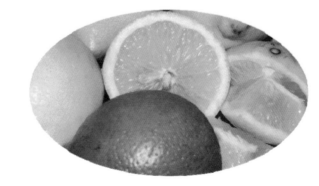

Other Flavours
Lemons
Limes
Honey
Garlic
Vanilla

1. Salmon with Lime and Honey

Serves 2

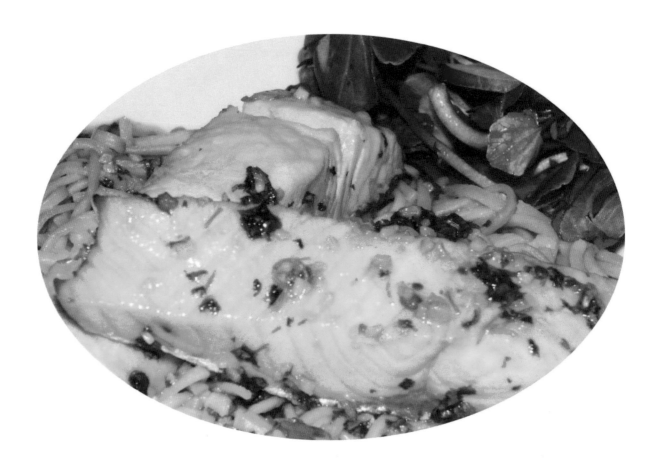

<u>Ingredients</u>

2 thick salmon fillets (or steaks)
25 g butter
1 clove garlic
1 lime
½ lemon
100ml white wine
1-2 teaspoons runny honey
Fresh coriander leaves (cilantro)

To serve: Noodles and Low-Ox salad (see page 26)

Preparation

1. Melt the butter in a frying pan. Add the crushed/minced garlic and fry for 1 minute.

2. Add the salmon (skin side down if using fillets).

3. Add the juice of the lime and half-lemon, wine and honey. Stir around the salmon.

4. Simmer 3-5 minutes, stirring occasionally, until the salmon is cooked through most of its thickness.

5. Turn the salmon, sprinkle in the chopped coriander/cilantro, turn off the heat and cover the pan.

6. Leave for 2 minutes to allow the residual heat in the pan to finish cooking the fish.

Using up Leftovers

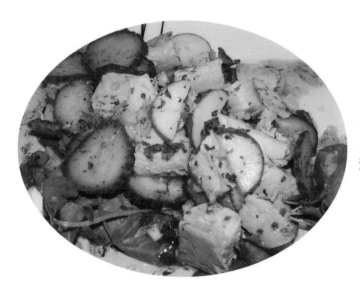

1. Make a cucumber salad: finely slice a cucumber, dice a white onion and put into a large, airtight jar. Add 4 teaspoons of caster sugar and pour in equal parts of olive oil and vinegar to cover the cucumber and onion. Add salt and pepper and 25g of finely chopped dill.

2. Shake well and serve with the cold salmon, watercress and crusty white bread. Garnish with radish slices. The Pink Salad Dressing on page 27 also goes well with this salad.

2. Trout with Apple Stuffing

Serves 2

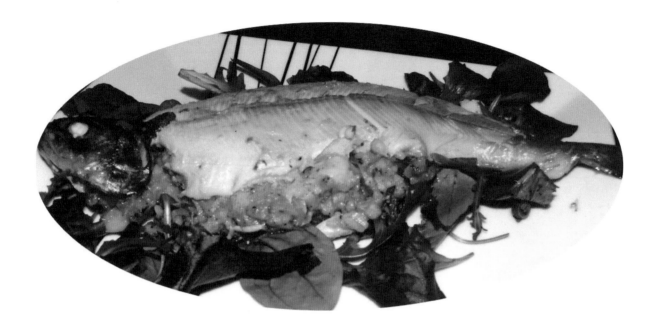

<u>Ingredients</u>

2 trout – cleaned

25g butter

1 white onion

1 Bramley apple

25g breadcrumbs

Juice of ½ lemon

1 teaspoon fresh lemon thyme

1 teaspoon fresh parsley

White pepper

Olive oil

Preparation

1. Melt the butter in a frying pan.

2. Dice the onion and fry until soft.

3. Core and dice the apple, and add to the onion. Fry for 1 minute.

4. Add the lemon juice, lemon thyme, parsley and a sprinkling of pepper, and mix well.

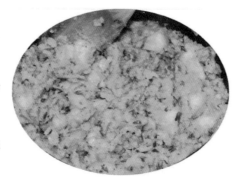

5. Fill the cavity of each trout with the stuffing and secure the opening with wooden cocktail sticks.

6. Brush the skin of the fish with olive oil and grill or bake 5-8 minutes each side until cooked (the eye will turn white and the flesh will flake).

7. Serve with low-ox salad or vegetable risotto.

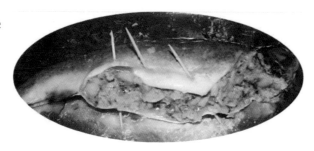

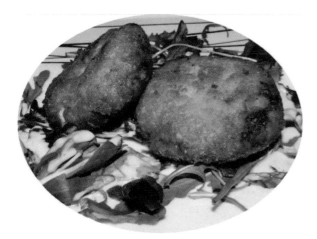

Using up leftovers

Flake the fish, mix with the stuffing and form into patties. Coat the fishcakes with flour, beaten egg then breadcrumbs and deep fry. Serve with lettuce leaves, vinaigrette and warmed crusty white bread.

3. Cod in a Garlic, Parsley and White Wine Sauce

Serves 2

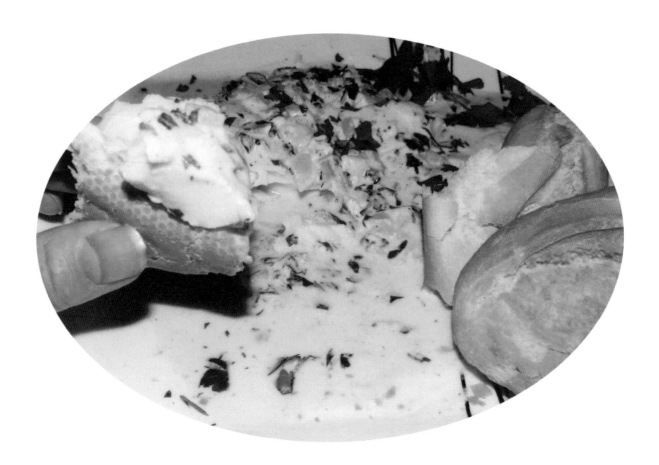

<u>Ingredients</u>

2 white fish steaks or fillets

1 white onion

6 garlic cloves (less if you prefer a milder flavour)

150ml dry white wine

300ml sour cream

2 teaspoons fresh parsley

Preparation

1. Finely dice the onion and crush the garlic, then fry until the onion is soft.

2. Add the wine and bubble until the alcohol has evaporated (the smell will become less pungent).

3. Take off the heat and stir in the sour cream.

4. Return to the heat, let the sauce bubble and add the fish. Turn the heat down to a gentle simmer, cover and cook for 5-10 minutes, depending on the thickness of your fish pieces, until the fish is just cooked.

5. Chop the parsley and add the majority to the pan, saving a small amount to sprinkle over the final plate.

6. Serve with warm, crusty, white buttered bread.

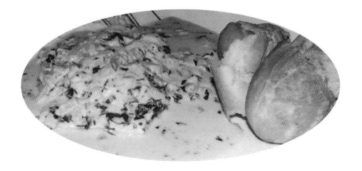

Using up Leftovers

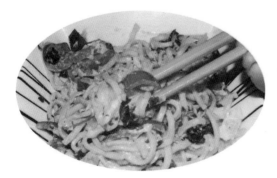

Stir fry noodles, onion, garlic and red peppers, and a few spoonfuls of the sauce. Add a handful of chopped fresh parsley leaves and flaked fish, fry for 30 seconds, and serve.

4. Chicken and Pesto Pasta

Serves 4

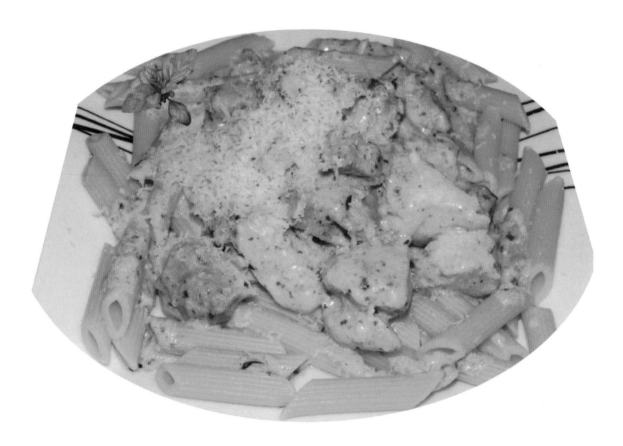

<u>Ingredients</u>

1 white onion

Sunflower oil

450g chicken breasts

225g thick cut roast ham or roast smoked gammon

3 teaspoons pesto

300ml sour cream

1 teaspoon cornflour

Serve with: Pasta and Parmesan cheese

Preparation

1. Dice the onion, and cube the chicken and ham/gammon, making the ham pieces approximately half the size of the chicken pieces.

2. Fry the onion until soft, then add the chicken and brown the meat.

3. Meanwhile, put the pasta in a pan with boiling water, stir, and leave to cook.

4. Add the ham or gammon to the chicken and onion, and cook, stirring for approximately 10 minutes until the chicken is cooked through.

5. Add the pesto to the chicken and ham, and stir in.

6. Take off the heat and stir in the sour cream. Return to heat.

7. Mix the cornflour with a little cold water, add to the pan and bubble for 2-3 minutes until thickened.

8. Serve over the cooked, drained pasta and grate parmesan over the dish.

9. Add a couple of basil leaves as garnish and serve with a low-ox salad.

Using Up Leftovers

Use the chicken and ham sauce as the filling for a pie – see recipe on page 16.

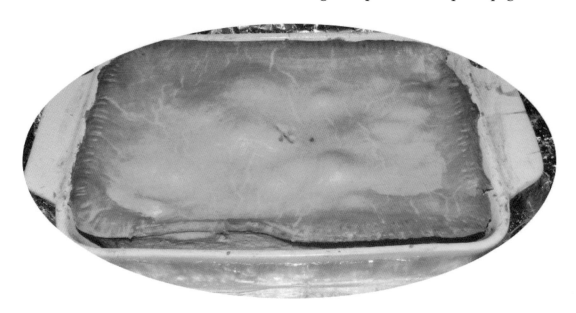

5. Lemon Chicken

Serves 2

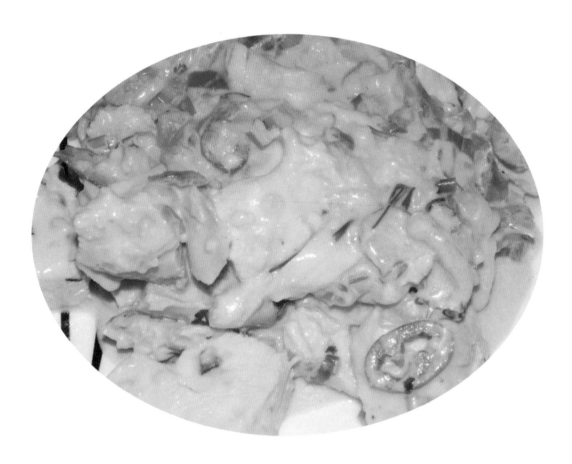

<u>Ingredients</u>

1 onion

2 cloves garlic

2 chicken breasts

1 red pepper

4 spring onions

1-2 green chillies

Juice of 1 lemon

1 teaspoon honey

100 ml sour cream

1 teaspoon coriander leaf (cilantro)

Preparation

1. Dice the onion and crush or mince the garlic, then fry until soft.

2. Cube the chicken breasts, add to the pan and brown the meat.

3. Slice the red pepper and chop the spring onions, and add to the pan. Stir.

4. Slice the green chillies, add to the pan and stir.

5. Add the lemon juice and honey. Stir well.

6. Cook 5-10 minutes until the chicken and vegetables are cooked through.

7. Add the sour cream and stir in, then the coriander leaf (cilantro).

8. Serve with white rice, noodles or pasta.

Using up Leftovers

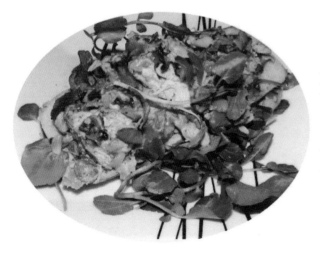

1. Reheat the chicken and sauce carefully yet thoroughly, so the chicken is heated through but the pieces stay whole.

2. Lightly toast ciabatta, sprinkle watercress over the bread, then top with the lemon chicken.

6. Mango and Lime Chicken

Serves 2

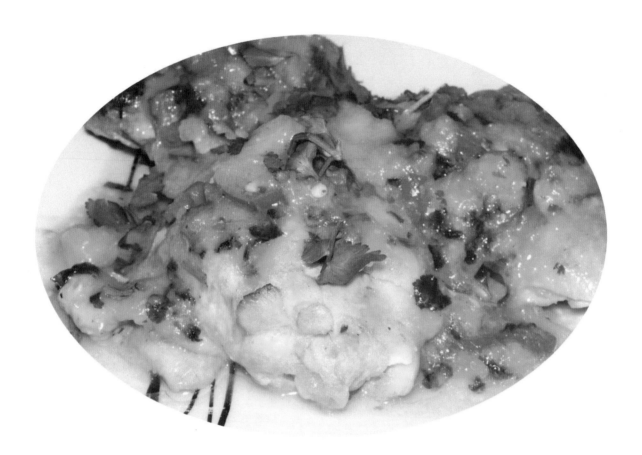

<u>Ingredients</u>

2 large chicken breasts or quarters

1 very ripe mango

Juice of 1 lime

Juice of ½ lemon

2 red chillies

1 teaspoon coriander leaf (cilantro)

Preparation

1. Pre-heat the oven to 220°C/425°F.

2. Put the chicken pieces into a deep baking dish.

3. Squeeze the juice of the lime and half lemon over the chicken.

4. Halve the mango, scoop and scrape out the flesh into a bowl. Crush it with a fork, then spoon this purée over the chicken.

5. Slice the chillies and scatter them over the chicken, along with most of the chopped coriander.

6. Cover the dish with foil and bake for 30 minutes.

7. Uncover, turn the chicken, baste, then bake another 30 minutes until the chicken is cooked through.

8. Serve, scattered with the remaining coriander leaves, with noodles or rice and low-ox salad.

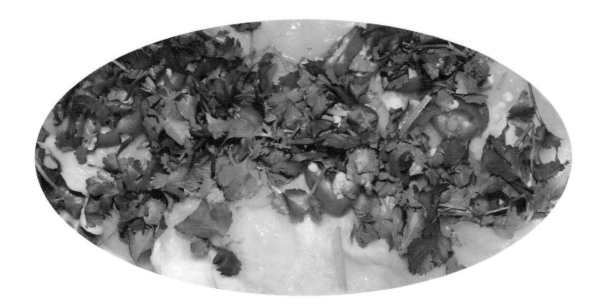

Using Up Leftovers

Dice the cold chicken, mix with mayonnaise and 2-3 teaspoons of the mango and lime sauce and serve with lightly toasted sourdough bread or ciabatta.

7. Chicken and Ham Pie

Serves 4

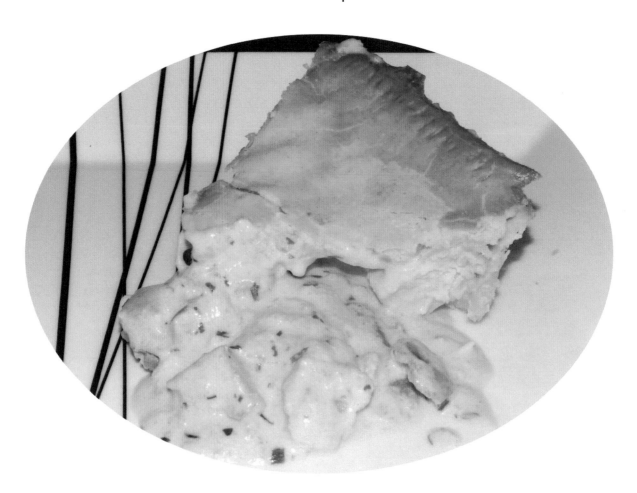

Ingredients

For the Filling:

1 white onion
Sunflower oil
450g chicken breasts/pieces
225g thick cut roast ham or roast
smoked gammon
3 teaspoons Dijon mustard
300ml sour cream
1 teaspoon fresh tarragon

For the Pastry:

450g plain flour
2 teaspoons baking powder
½ teaspoon salt
125g butter
1 egg yolk
100-150ml cold water
1 egg
Extra flour

Preparation

1. First prepare the pastry by adding the flour, baking powder, salt, butter and egg yolk to a food processor. Use the cutting blades and pulse function to process until the mixture looks like fine breadcrumbs. Alternatively cube the butter and rub it into the dry ingredients, adding the egg yolk afterwards.

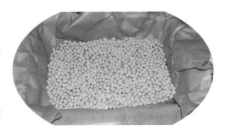

2. Add the water a bit at a time until the dough comes together in a ball. Wrap this in cling film and put in the fridge for an hour to chill.

3. Turn on the oven to 180°C/350°F to pre-heat.

4. Dice the onion, and cube the chicken and ham/gammon, making the ham pieces approximately half the size of the chicken pieces.

5. Fry the onion until soft, then add chicken and brown.

6. Add the ham or gammon, and cook, stirring for approximately 10 minutes until the chicken is cooked through.

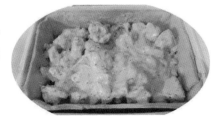

7. Add the mustard to the chicken and ham, and stir.

8. Take off the heat and stir in the sour cream and chopped tarragon. Return to the heat.

9. Mix the cornflour with a little cold water, add to the pan and bubble for 2-3 minutes until thickened. Turn off the heat and allow to cool.

11. Grease your pie dish, roll out approximately 2/3 of your chilled pastry on a floured surface until it is large enough to cover the base and sides of the dish. Use the rolling pin to transfer it to the dish and gently press it down inside against the base and sides, then prick the base several times with a fork.

12. Trim the excess pastry, line the pie with greaseproof paper, and cover the base with rice or dried beans. Bake in the oven for 10 minutes, then discard the paper and beans, and allow the pie base to cool.

13. Add the filling to the pie base.

14. Roll out the rest of the pastry to a size large enough to cover the top of your dish. Beat the egg and brush the rim of your pie base. Use your rolling pin to pick up your pie lid and drape it over the top of the pie. Trim off any excess pastry. (Leftover tip: Use up the trimmed pastry to make jam tarts).

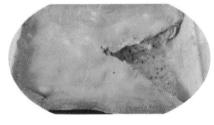

14. Crimp the edges with a fork, cut a small cross into the centre of the lid to allow steam to vent and brush the top of the pie with beaten egg.

15. Put in the oven and bake for 30-35 minutes until golden brown.

8. Pork Steaks with a Mustard and Apple Sauce

Serves 2

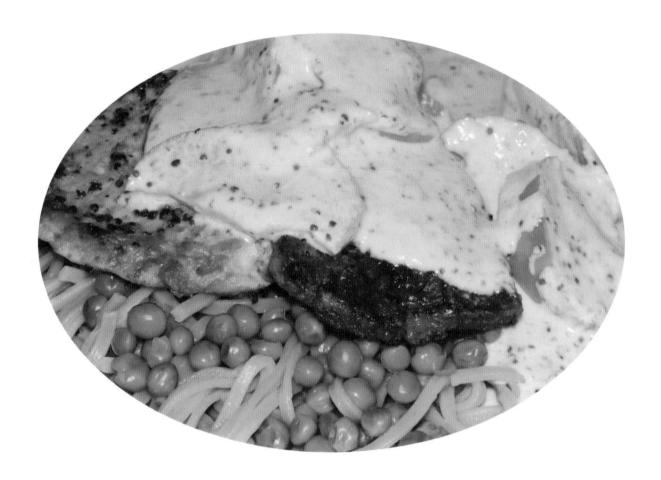

<u>Ingredients</u>

2-4 pork steaks, depending on size

Wholegrain mustard

250ml sour cream

250ml white wine

1 apple

Noodles and peas to serve

Preparation

1. Rub ¼ teaspoon of mustard into each side of each pork steak. Grill for 10-20 minutes, depending on thickness, and turning until cooked through, taking care not to overcook.

2. Meanwhile, prepare the sauce.

3. Core and slice the apple and poach in the wine for about 5 minutes until the alcohol has evaporated and the liquid reduced.

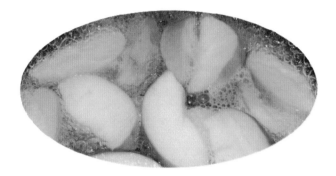

4. Remove from the heat and stir in the sour cream. Return to the heat and allow to bubble.

5. Remove from the heat and stir in 3 teaspoons of mustard. Return to the heat and allow to bubble. Reduce the heat and simmer.

6. Cook the noodles and peas and serve with the pork steaks. Spoon the apples and sauce over the dish.

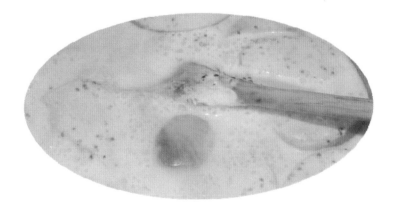

9. Smoked Gammon, Sauerkraut and Bread Dumplings

Serves 4

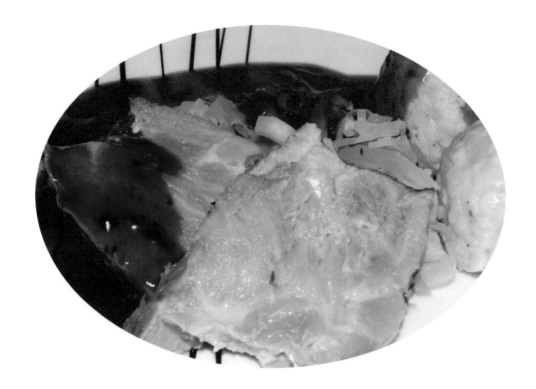

<u>Ingredients</u>

Smoked gammon joint
Sunflower oil
2 beef stock cubes
Jar of sauerkraut
Pinch of caraway seeds

<u>For the Bread Dumplings:</u>
4 stale bread buns/slices
150ml milk
25g butter
2 rashers streaky bacon
1 white onion
2 eggs
Salt and pepper
Plain flour
(You can also flavour the dumplings with chopped, fresh herbs or caraway seeds)

Preparation

1. Pre-heat the oven to 200°C/400°F. Rub the gammon joint with the oil, crumbled stock cubes and pinch of caraway seeds.

2. Put on to a roasting tray then into oven for 45 minutes.

3. Turn, baste and bake for a further 45 minutes until the meat is cooked through.

4. To make the bread dumplings, first use a food processor to turn the bread into crumbs, then put into a mixing bowl. Alternatively, grate the bread slices into crumbs.

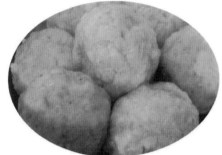

5. Melt the butter, add the milk and warm through, then add to the breadcrumbs and mix well.

6. Dice the bacon and onion, melt a small knob of butter, and fry until the bacon is cooked and onion is soft. Add mixture to breadcrumbs and mix well.

7. Add the eggs, salt and plenty of black pepper and mix well.

8. Shape breadcrumb mixture into dumplings, dip and roll each one in a dish of plain flour, then roll them in your hands again to a smooth, round shape.

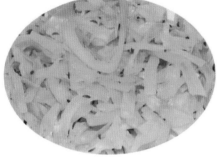

9. Bring a large pan of water to the boil, add salt, turn the heat down to simmer, and carefully place each dumpling into the pan with a slotted spoon.

10. Simmer for 20 minutes, then remove the dumplings from the pan with the slotted spoon, and drain in a colander.

11. Spoon your desired amount of sauerkraut into small saucepan and add a small sprinkle of caraway seeds. Gently heat through, for about 5 minutes.

12. Serve with gravy and mild German mustard.

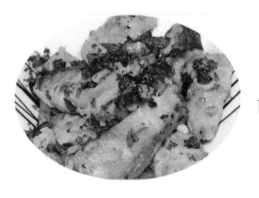

Using Up Leftovers:

Dice an onion and slice a deseeded red chilli. Fry in butter and sunflower oil until soft. Slice the bread dumplings into chips (the thinner they are, the crispier). Chop slices of gammon and add to the pan. Fry until browned and serve with salad.

10. Steak with Dijon Mustard Sauce

Serves 2-4

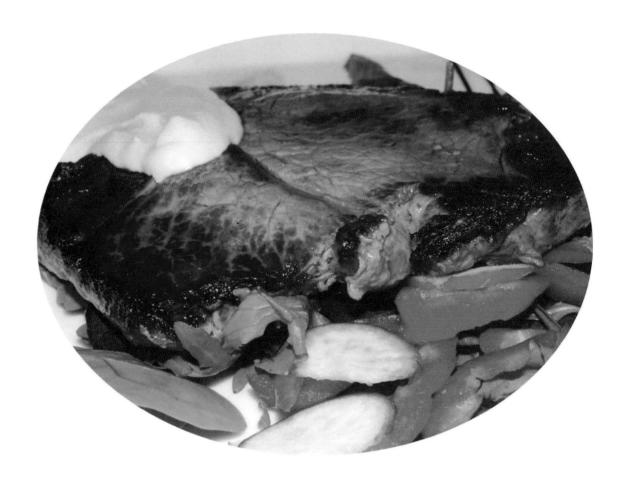

Ingredients

1 steak per person, of your desired cut

300ml crème fraiche

2 teaspoons Dijon mustard

Serve with: Low-ox salad and warm, crusty white bread or

Red cabbage and risotto.

Preparation

1. Take the steaks out of the fridge ahead of time to let them reach room temperature before cooking.

2. Heat the oil in a frying pan, then fry 2-5 minutes each side depending on the thickness of your steak and whether you prefer your steak rare, medium or well done.

3. Check the steak is cooked to your preference by touch – rare: soft, medium: bouncy, well done: firm.

3. Season the steak, turn off the heat, and put on one side to rest for a maximum of 5 minutes to allow the juices to be reabsorbed into the meat fibres and tenderise the beef.

3. Meanwhile, pour the crème fraiche into a saucepan and heat through.

4. Take off the heat and add the mustard. Mix well and return to the heat.

5. Heat through until bubbling. Turn heat to very low until the steaks have rested.

6. Serve.

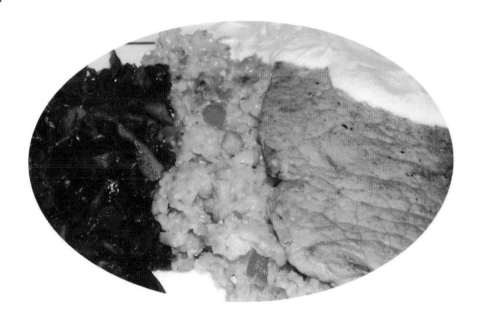

Using up leftovers

Slice steak thinly, mix with the sauce and serve with lettuce in wraps.

11. Risotto
Serves 4

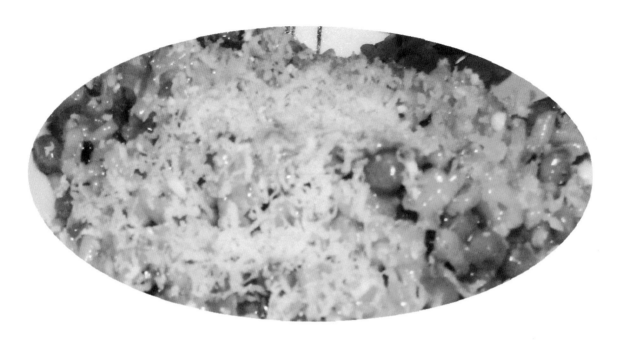

<u>Ingredients</u>

225g risotto rice

2 rashers thick, smoked bacon

2 anchovy fillets

1 white onion

4 cloves garlic

4 radishes

1 red pepper

1 courgette (zucchini)

200ml peas

200 ml white wine

3 chicken stock cubes

Fresh herbs – chives, parsley and thyme

Salt and white pepper

Parmesan cheese

Preparation

1. Fry the diced onion and crushed garlic in oil in a large pot for 2 minutes until soft.

2. Dice the anchovies and bacon and add to the pan. Fry until browned.

3. Add the chopped vegetables.

4. Stir well.

5. Add the rice and the wine and stir well.

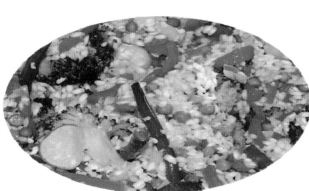

6. Make up approx. 200ml hot stock with the stock cubes.

7. Add a little to the risotto, stirring well.

8. Once the liquid has been absorbed, add a little more and stir.

9. Keep adding in this way until the rice is soft and cooked. If you run out of stock, use hot water until you have enough liquid to properly cook the rice.

10. Chop the herbs and soak in a little hot water for 5-10 minutes, then add to the dish at the end, with salt and pepper.

11. Turn off the heat, cover the pan and rest for two minutes.

12. Serve sprinkled with parmesan cheese, either on its own or as an accompaniment to fish or meat dishes.

Using up leftovers

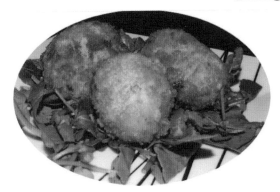

Add grated mozzarella to the cold risotto and form into 1-inch diameter balls, cover with flour, beaten egg, then breadcrumbs and deep fry. Serve with salad as a snack for lunch or as an accompaniment to steak, chicken breasts or fish.

12. Low-Ox Salad

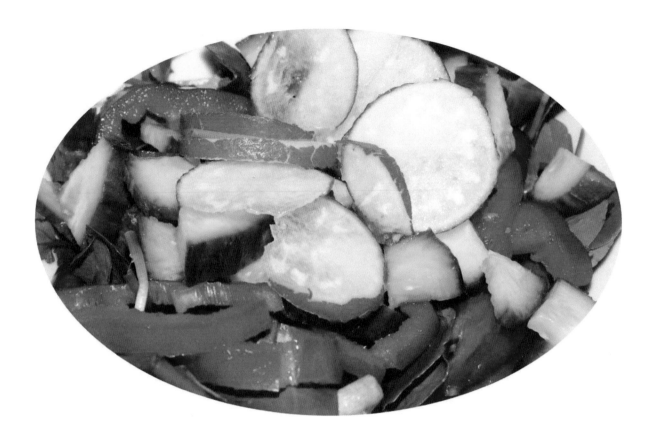

Ingredients

Watercress

Red pepper

Cucumber

Radish

Preparation

1. Chop peppers, cucumber and radish.
2. Add to watercress in a salad bowl.

13. Pink Salad Dressing

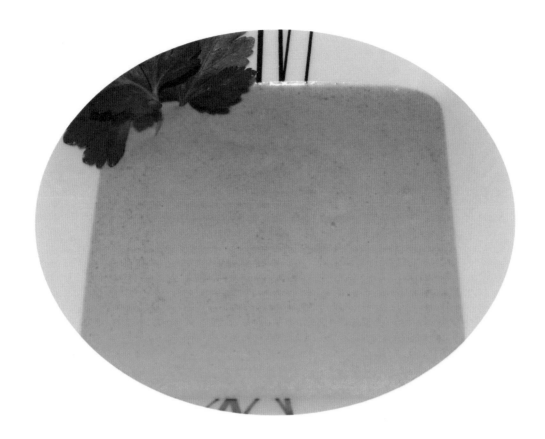

Ingredients

4 tablespoons mayonnaise

4 tablespoons tomato ketchup

Juice of ½ lemon

Pinch cayenne pepper

Preparation

1. Spoon mayonnaise into a bowl and stir well (this avoids lumps in the finished sauce).

2. Add ketchup and stir in, then add the lemon juice and pinch of cayenne (more if you like a kick!).

3. Mix well.

14. Vinaigrette

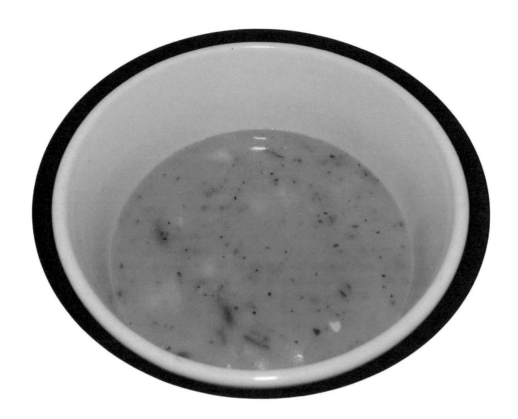

Ingredients

1 shallot
1 garlic clove
1 teaspoon Dijon mustard
2 teaspoons honey
1 teaspoon fresh herbs – rosemary, sage and thyme
Salt and pepper
2 tablespoons white wine vinegar
4 tablespoons extra virgin olive oil

Preparation

1. Finely dice the shallot and garlic clove and mix in a jar with the mustard, honey, herbs, salt and pepper.

2. Add the vinegar and oil and shake well.

15. German Meat Salad

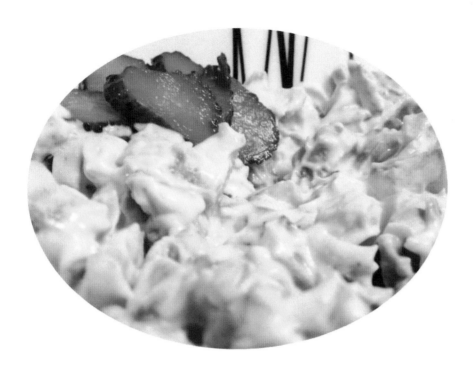

Ingredients

Cold smoked gammon and ham

Equal amount of sweet-and-sour pickled gherkins

Mayonnaise

Preparation

1. Finely dice the meat.

2. Roughly chop the gherkins to a similar size.

3. Add enough mayonnaise to cover the ingredients.

4. Mix well.

Serve with crusty bread, cold meats and low-ox salad.

16. Vanilla Panna Cotta

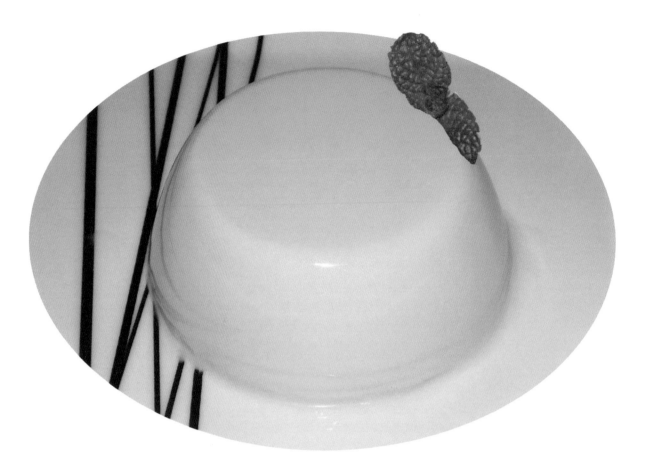

<u>Ingredients</u>

300 ml double cream

300 ml milk

100g caster sugar

2 teaspoons vanilla extract

4 gelatine leaves (platinum grade)

Preparation

1. Put the gelatine leaves into a bowl of cold water to soak for 10 minutes.

2. Grease 6 small pudding moulds or ramekin dishes.

2. Put the cream and milk into a heavy bottomed saucepan and bring to the boil.

3. Reduce the heat, add the sugar and vanilla extract, and stir until the sugar is dissolved.

4. When the gelatine has finished soaking, remove it from the water with clean fingers and add to the cream mixture.

5. Stir until dissolved.

6. Pour the mixture into the greased moulds/ramekins and allow to cool, then refrigerate overnight.

7. To serve, carefully dip the bowl into hot water for 1 second, then turn out on to a damp plate. Position the panna cotta, then garnish with a sprig of mint.

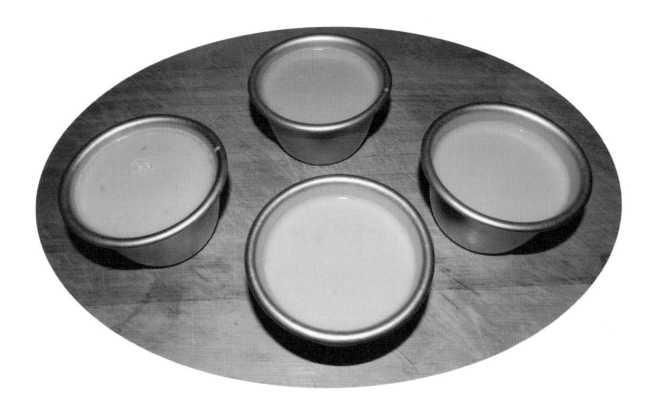

17. Lemon Pancakes

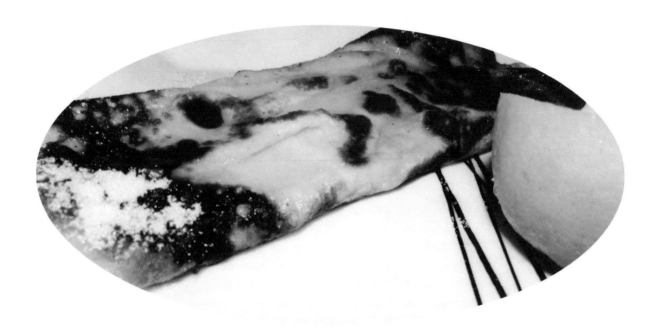

<u>Ingredients</u>

125g self-raising flour

1 tablespoon caster sugar

2 eggs

300ml milk

Pinch nutmeg

Butter

Lemon

Caster sugar

Preparation

1. Sift the flour into a bowl, crack in the eggs, 50 ml of the milk, and the sugar and nutmeg.

2. Whisk to combine (either by hand or with a food mixer).

3. Continue to beat as you slowly add more milk until you get the consistency of double cream, which coats the back of a spoon.

4. Heat a knob of butter in a small frying pan.

5. Pour in enough batter to coat the base of the pan and cook approx. 30 seconds until the bottom is golden brown – use a fish slice to check underneath.

6. Flip – either with a fish slice or by tossing – then cook a further 30 seconds.

7. Serve, squeeze lemon juice the top and sprinkle with sugar.

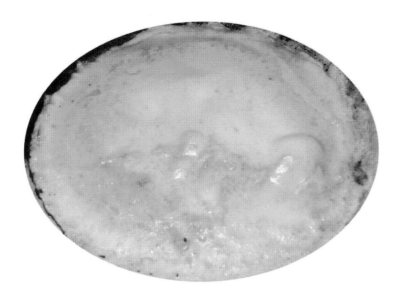

Using Up Leftovers

The uncooked pancake mixture will keep in the fridge for a few days to be cooked when required.

References:

http://emedicine.medscape.com/article/2182757-overview

http://nof.org/foods

http://www.coreonehealth.com/oxalates-and-their-role-in-fibromyalgia-syndrome

http://www.dailymail.co.uk/health/article-2174474/The-GP-gave-fruit-veg-cure-aches-pains.html

http://www.litholink.com/downloads/stone_lowoxalatediet.pdf

http://www.lowoxalate.info/food_lists/alph_lod_food_chart.pdf

http://www.upmc.com/patients-visitors/education/nutrition/Pages/low-oxalate-diet.aspx

http://www.urologyweb.com/calcium-stones/

http://www.whfoods.com/genpage.php?tname=george&dbid=48

For more information on the full range of Minna Rose's cookbooks, including links for the main retailer sites, please go to Minna's website: www.minnarose.com

If you would like to contact Minna or join Minna's mailing list to be kept updated of news, upcoming releases and special offers, please go to: www.minnarose.com/contact-minna-rose

Made in the USA
Columbia, SC
01 May 2018